Eat
This
Because
I
Said
So

BY:
Chris Kitchen, Bev Hansen, Jane Thiel

Order this book online at www.trafford.com/08-0385
or email orders@trafford.com

Most Trafford titles are also available at major online book retailers.

Note for Librarians: A cataloguing record for this book is available from Library
and Archives Canada at www.collectionscanada.ca/amicus/index-e.html

ISBN: 978-1-4251-4850-8

*We at Trafford believe that it is the responsibility of us all, as both individuals
and corporations, to make choices that are environmentally and socially sound.
You, in turn, are supporting this responsible conduct each time you purchase a
Trafford book, or make use of our publishing services. To find out how you are
helping, please visit www.trafford.com/responsiblepublishing.html*

*Our mission is to efficiently provide the world's finest, most comprehensive
book publishing service, enabling every author to experience success.
To find out how to publish your book, your way, and have it available
worldwide, visit us online at www.trafford.com/10510*

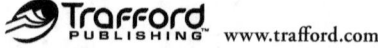 www.trafford.com

North America & international
toll-free: 1 888 232 4444 (USA & Canada)
phone: 250 383 6864 ♦ fax: 250 383 6804 ♦ email: info@trafford.com

The United Kingdom & Europe
phone: +44 (0)1865 722 113 ♦ local rate: 0845 230 9601
facsimile: +44 (0)1865 722 868 ♦ email: info.uk@trafford.com

10 9 8 7 6 5 4 3 2 1

Dedicated to my brother Mike. I admire his
courage to take a chance.
Chris

TABLE OF CONTENTS

PREFACE

The authors (Chris, Bev and Jane) are NOT doctors, nutritionists, or nurses. We are just average people who have discovered the secret to eating healthy and taking control of our weight.

This book will help YOU take control of YOUR healthy lifestyle as well. We share with you the knowledge we have learned to make good choices in the food you put into your mouth. We have included bits of humor to help you along the way (remember—laughing is an excellent exercise!).

Most importantly—YOU have the chance to determine how to script the rest of your life. What's past is past, what's done is done, what's important is what's to come. You can choose to keep doing what you've always done (just don't expect different results) or you can choose to write a new chapter for a new, healthier, YOU!

This is a cookbook, but unlike any cookbook you've ever used before. Following the information in this book will enable you to create a new—healthy—you. Enjoy!

INTRODUCTION

OK, here's the deal. You fall into one of three categories of humans:

1. You *can* eat anything you want, but if you do you'll end-up being one of those 500+ pound people that will have to be lifted out of their home by a crane through the picture window.
2. You *can* eat anything you want, but you're still a 98 pound weakling who gets sand kicked in his face at the beach.
3. You *can* eat anything you want and you stay slim/slender with no ill effects.

If you fall into category 1 or 2 this book is for you. If you fall into category 3 the rest of the world hates you and wishes you could spend at least *some* time in category 1 or 2 so you can experience what the rest of us suffer with. This information is not for category 3-type people, unless they prepare food for someone in category 1 or 2.

This book is targeted to those who want to change and/or maintain their weight. Essentially this book is about:

EATING HEALTHY

That's it! The focus of this book is NOT about dieting, about losing weight, or about gaining weight—although there is information here that will help you do that. The focus is about eating healthy. The cool thing is, however, when you eat healthy food, in the right proportion, you WILL lose weight or gain weight because you will find YOUR right weight!

There's a computer term those wacky computer geeks came up with years ago. It's called GIGO (pronounced "gee-go"). It stands for "Garbage In, Garbage Out." What it means is: if you program the wrong information (garbage) into the computer, you will get useless information (garbage) out of the program. We sometimes think that should apply to our bodies as well. The problem is, our bodies are sneaky. If we ingest garbage (large greasy fries, candy bars, too many margaritas) our body has a tendency to retain the garbage...as fat! Kind of like—GIGS—let's pronounce that "geesh" (I know it doesn't look like that but, geesh!) "Garbage In, Garbage Stays." Of course, some people want to GAIN weight and think eating all that garbage will help them pack on the pounds—all they get is a bad complexion out of the deal.

Nobody said controlling your weight would be easy (at least not for MOST of the world's population... we're not going to talk about those category 3 people any more). It's not an impossible task, it's just not easy (until you get the hang of it that is). This book will teach you about:

- Food—information about each of the food categories (fats, dairy, proteins, carbohydrates, fruits and vegetables)
- Your body—you have to know how your body operates before you can efficiently fuel it. You have to know what it needs before you start filling it up.
- Other tid-bits of information that the authors feel you should know.

In addition to all the above, there are two weeks of healthy-eating menu plans (minus a day "off" for healthy-eating behavior each week). Recipes are included for those items marked with an asterisk on the menu plans (oh yeah, this is also a cookbook!).

Your mother probably nagged you about several things while you were growing up. If you've forgotten, or were never told, here's a reminder -

- SIT-UP STRAIGHT! Don't slouch or your back will freeze that way!
- EAT! At least 5 or 6 times a day!

- EXERCISE! Start with 15 minutes of walking. Get off your bum!
- SLEEP! You need 7-9 hours, not a whole day's worth!
- TAKE YOUR VITAMINS! Get a good, food-derived vitamin and take your Omega (fish oil) too! (At least you don't have to drink cod liver oil like we did, back in the old days...believe me, the pill is easier to swallow.)

Let's expound on each of these bits of wisdom:

SIT-UP STRAIGHT
Improving your posture (standing and sitting with your back straight) will do more than get your mother off your back. Many aches and pains can be eliminated with good posture. It also makes you look better (even thinner!).

EAT
You know that you have to put fuel in your engine before your car runs...you also have to fuel your body. If you're trying to lose weight one of the functions of the body that will help you is your metabolism. Your metabolism helps you to turn the food into energy. It can be high (which is good) or low (not so good). We'll delve into this subject more later. If you eat several small meals a day your metabolism will be revved-up and continue helping you—and you won't feel so deprived by not eating.

On the other hand, if you're trying to gain weight, eating several meals a day will help you get all those calories in without feeling too full. Pretty cool how that works, don't you think?

EXERCISE
I know, I know, we hate hearing that 8-letter E word—but you know you need it. The thing is, you don't have to invest in any equipment, just MOVE! In the case of

exercise, the little things count: take the stairs, park farther away from the mall (or the restaurant!), turn on the tunes and dance while you do the dishes. There are many—small—ways you can incorporate this into your day.

SLEEP
Scientists have been studying this subject and have determined that you are more able to lose weight if you get 7-9 hours of sleep a night. When you deprive yourself of sleep, your body tells you you're hungry so you're more likely to eat. So turn off the TV and the computer and get those z's. Why? Because I said so!

TAKE YOUR VITAMINS
We no longer get the proper nutrition in our food like our ancestors did. Because of that it is a good idea to take supplemental vitamins. Make sure, however, that you are taking good food-based vitamins. A good way to tell if your vitamins can be absorbed by your body is to put one in a glass of water. It should dissolve—if it does not, it will probably go through your system without any effect.

FOOD

All food falls into one of the following categories:
- Fats
- Dairy
- Proteins
- Carbohydrates
- Fruits & Vegetables

To control your weight, you need to eat the proper amount of each of these categories. You can't just eliminate all fats or all carbohydrates...or load-up on them. Your body needs each of the categories to remain healthy. The trick then, is determine HOW MUCH of each category you need to consume.

FATS

Fat has a bad rep. Just the mere mention of it makes people cringe! Lots of things can be done with fat: gain it, lose it, cook with it and cry about it! What we don't realize is: NOT ALL FAT IS BAD. In fact, your brain needs fatty acids to function (gives new meaning to the term fathead). Without going into detail, fats that occur naturally in a product (i.e. fat in lean meat, butter, milk, nuts, etc.) are not bad, in moderation. What we need to avoid is processed, man-made, trans fats (ie: the fat in margarine, potato chips, greasy french fries, etc.).

Unsaturated Fats are filled with Essential Fatty Acids. Essential is the key word—essential for many important processes in the body like energy and hormone production, to name a few. Good sources of unsaturated fats are avocados, olive oil, nuts and seeds.
We don't want too much of a good thing here, though. The goal is to eat foods that are low in fat (not necessarily fat-free) and packed full of good nutrients.

DAIRY

According to the National Dairy Council, Americans

tend to be overfed and obese—but severely undernourished! Where can we get good nourishment? DAIRY. Dairy products are packed full of essential vitamins and minerals: calcium, potassium, protein, and vitamins A, B-12, and D to mention a few! Including low-fat or fat-free dairy products in your diet can actually speed weight loss.

Dairy products are derived from milk and include: milk, yogurt, cheese, butter, and ice cream.

Yogurt is packed full of live cultures called "acidophilus". Acidophilus is a group of probiotics (or healthy bacteria) that aid in healthy digestion. The health of our intestinal tracts can play a huge role in the function of our immune system.

Butter is an excellent source of vitamin A, trace minerals, and essential fatty acids. Always use butter rather than margarine and vegetable oil spreads. Some people on a low-fat diet avoid butter all together but the good news is they don't have to! About 15% of the fats in butter are not stored but are used by the body for energy—so start buttering-up, people!

Ice cream—the sinful delight? No! You don't need to go buy a size bigger jean if you indulge in ice cream—but you must make the right choices. Now, we aren't saying sit in front of the TV watching "Gone With the Wind" with a carton of Triple Fudge Caramel with Cherries and a box of tissues. You can make GOOD ice cream choices that are tasty too! Choose a low-fat or fat-free ice cream and top with fruit to get the bang for your buck in nutritional value.

PROTEINS

A well-balanced diet includes adequate servings of protein. Protein builds muscle and muscle burns more calories than fat. However, the amount of recommended daily protein depends on your age and health. For most adults 2 to 3 servings will meet the daily needs.

The following are recommended serving sizes:
- 2 to 3 ounces of lean meat, poultry, or fish
- 1/2 cup beans
- 1 egg
- 2 tablespoons peanut butter
- 1 ounce cheese

These can be visualized as the following:
- 1 ounce of meat—pack of matches
- 3 ounces of meat—bar of soap
- 2 ounces of fish—checkbook
- 1 ounce of cheese—4 dice

SUGAR AND CARBOHYDRATES

Whoa! What are we doing here? Mixing two categories? No—the fact is, sugar is sucrose, and sucrose is a carbohydrate. The body turns carbohydrates into energy....so we need' em! The problem is we don't usually get them in the proper form, or amount.

Sugar has a bad reputation when it comes to weight loss. We think that we can just cut out all sugar and we'll be skinny with great teeth—right? Wrong. While some sugars aren't good for you (like the white granulated sugar you spoon on your already-sweetened cereal), we can't just cut out ALL sugar. To do that you would practically have to quit eating altogether—sugar is found in almost every food.

As far as carbohydrates, remember: carbs are not a no-no! Carbs give you energy and, for you diabetics, can help stabilize blood sugar levels. Also, good carbs are full of fiber so they can help make you feel fuller faster. (hint, hint: WEIGHT LOSS!!)

So—how do we know which carbs are good and which are bad?

GOOD CARBS = HIGH IN FIBER!
>   fruits, veggies, whole grain breads,
>   beans, nuts

BAD CARBS = WHITE! WHITE! WHITE!
>   white breads, white pastas,
>   white sugars

To add sweetness go for the honey or molasses. Or, better yet, eat something naturally sweet—like an apple or watermelon. You don't have to totally abandon all sugar to control your healthy weight, just look at healthy alternatives to getting that sweet taste we all love. So what about sugar substitutes? Avoid artificial sweeteners—go for the natural instead.

HONEY—Honey works for more than just sweetening. It has healing properties as well. Honey can sooth sore throats and calm upset stomachs. Honey is rich in antioxidants and microbe-fighting effects. As with other carbs—dark is better than light. Buckwheat honey has been prescribed by some doctors to limit children's coughing. CAUTION: Children younger than 12 months should not be fed honey since it can cause botulism in infants.

STEVIA—Stevia can be found in most health food stores. It is a non-caloric herb sweeter than sugar. It comes in many forms and is labeled as a "dietary supplement." Hey moms—stevia has been known to reduce cavities in kids!

FRUITS & VEGETABLES

I'm sure your mother told you to eat your vegetables to grow up strong and healthy—that's good advice! Fruits and vegetables should be included in everybody's diet to promote good health. Fruits and veggies have disease-fighting fiber, antioxidants, phytochemicals and vitamins. Antioxidants help defend against free radicals. (Note: This could get real technical, real quick! Think of it this way: free radicals are bad, antioxidants are good.)

Phytochemicals are non-nutrient chemicals found in plants that have been discovered to contain protective/disease-preventing compounds. (Again, this could be very technical—just know that phytochemicals are good things, they help your body stay healthy.)

The CDC (Center for Disease Control and Prevention) as well as the American Cancer Institute and other governmental organizations suggest a minimum of 5 servings of fruits and vegetables a day. Other organizations are suggesting not just 5, but at least 5—the more, the better!

The benefits of adding fruits and vegetables:
- Lowers the risk of heart disease
- Lowers blood pressure
- Lowers cholesterol
- Prevents certain cancers
- Aids digestion and triggers regular bowel movements
- Helps feed the eyes with the nutrients needed to keep seeing clearly

To get the most bang-for-your-buck, go for variety—dark-green leafy vegetables; yellow, orange and red fruits and vegetables; cooked tomatoes; and citrus fruits. Different fruits and vegetables help different parts of the body—go for the rainbow. Not only should fruits and/or vegetables be included with every meal—they make an excellent choice for a snack!

WORTH REPEATING

"Never eat more than you can lift."
- Miss Piggy

"You must do the thing you think you cannot do."
- Eleanor Roosevelt

"Rich, fatty foods are like destiny:
they too, shape our ends."
- Author Unknown

"Nothing tastes as good as being thin feels."
- Author Unknown

"When I buy cookies I eat just four and throw the rest
away. But first I spray them with Raid so I won't dig
them out of the garbage later. Be careful, though,
because that Raid doesn't really taste that bad."
- Janette Barber

"You've got to say, 'I think if I keep working at this and
want it badly enough I can have it.'
It's called perseverance."
- Lee Iacocca

"No diet will remove all the fat from your body because
the brain is entirely fat. Without a brain you might look
good, but all you can do is run for public office."
- George Bernard Shaw

YOUR BODY

To lose weight you have to expend more energy than you take in. In other words, you have to eat fewer calories than you burn. Sounds simple: right? You are probably saying to yourself, "Wait! There's one problem! How do I know how many calories I burn?"

The answer is in your Resting Metabolic Rate (RMR). In simple terms, the RMR is the amount of calories you burn to keep your vital organs functioning. By using the Harris Benedict Equation you will be able to figure out your RMR and your Target Caloric Weight Loss Zone. This zone gives you the maximum amount of calories you can eat and still lose weight!

The key to understanding your Target Caloric Weight Loss Zone is to first understand some of the basic principles of metabolism and how it's affecting your weight loss efforts.

As mentioned before, your Resting Metabolic Rate (RMR) is the amount of calories you burn at rest. In the past you were just playing a guessing game on how many calories you were burning in a day. How many times have you heard, "Eat 1200 calories a day and you will lose weight!" Okay, Great! Now why isn't that working? Let's think about this. How could caloric intake requirements be the same for all people? Why doesn't a simple reduction in calories work? The truth is, eating the <u>required</u> amount of calories for yourself is the key to weight control. While eating too many calories leads to weight gain, eating too <u>few</u> calories may slow your metabolic rate resulting in a weight gain or a plateau!

1200 calories may be too few for you—you may find that you're burning 1500 calories at rest! On the other hand, 1200 calories may be too much for you, actually leading to a gain of 1 pound (or more) a month! (3500 calories equals 1 pound. If you eat 117 calories a day more than you burn you will gain a pound a month.) By knowing your RMR and Target Caloric Weight Loss Zone you will have actual numbers that will lead to actual results!

By using the following equation you will be able to approximate your RMR and your Weight Loss Calorie Zone– WLCZ. (Again, 3500 calories = 1 pound, decreasing your calories by 500 a day will enable you to lose 1 pound a week—a good, sensible, level of weight loss.) These numbers will give you the tools you need to understand your own body and what it needs to succeed!

Harris Benedict Equation

Female RMR = 655 + (9.6 x weight in pounds x 0.455) + (1.8 x height in inches x 2.4) - (4.7 x age in years)

Male RMR = 66 + (13.7 x weight in lbs x 0.455) + (5 x height in inches x 2.4) - (6.8 x age in years)

WLCZ = (1.2 x RMR) - 500

Examples:

A 28 year old female weighing 150 pounds, standing 5'2" in height:
RMR = 655 + (9.6 x 150 x 0.455) + (1.8 x 62 x 2.4) - (4.7 x 28) = 1446.44
WLCZ = (1.2 x 1446.44) - 500 = 1235.73

This female can eat a maximum of approximately 1236 calories per day in order to lose 1 pound (1.5 to 2 lbs. with exercise!) per week.

A 28 year old male weighing 200 pounds, standing 6' in height:

RMR = 66 + (13.7 x 200 x 0.455) + (5 x 72 x 2.4) - (6.8 x 28) = 1986.3
WLCZ = (1.2 x 1986.3) - 500 = 1883.56

This male can eat a maximum of approximately 1884 calories per day in order to lose 1 pound (1.5 to 3 lbs. with exercise) per week.

Medically Supervised Zone:
We DO NOT recommend consuming less than 1000 calories per day without a doctor's recommendation. This zone is more often than not too low for most people. It is so important to get the nutrients your body needs and if your calorie intake is too low your metabolic rate will slow down. In return, your body perceives that it is starving and will hang onto every last calorie instead of burning it. Only under the direct supervision of a physician should you be in this zone!

WORTH REPEATING

"If you have formed the habit of checking on every new diet that comes along, you will find that, mercifully, they all blur together, leaving you with only one definite piece of information: french-fried potatoes are out."
- Jean Kerr

"The older you get, the tougher it is to lose weight because by then your body and your fat are really good friends."
- Author Unknown

"You're never beaten until you admit it."
- George S. Patton

"You have to stay in shape. My grandmother – she started walking five miles a day when she was 60. She's 97 today and we don't know where the heck she is."
- Ellen Degeneres

"Inside some of us is a thin person struggling to get out, but they can usually be sedated with a few pieces of chocolate cake."
- Author Unknown

NOW WHAT?

Here are a few tricks & tips to help you if weight loss is your goal.

- DRINK WATER—exclude any and all soda from your diet if you can, or at least start drinking less of it. When looking at water—all is not the same. Be sure to read the labels on the bottled waters—some can be loaded with calories! If your water at home is filtered, drink up! FIJI® brand water is also an excellent choice—it has silica, calcium and magnesium in it and it has been shown to help with weight loss.

  If you're just starting your healthy weight program do a water flush. Drink it all day! Start with it right away when you get up and end with it right before you go to bed. Also, before and after each meal and snack. You'll be surprised how different you feel after about 3-5 days of that (of course, you will be going to the bathroom a lot—there seems to be a downside to most everything sometimes!).

  Even after the water flush, drink a glass of water before each meal—it will help you feel full sooner.

- SERVING SIZE—make sure you understand HOW MUCH a serving of your food choice is. Most packaged foods (whole grain bread, low-fat ice cream, etc.) have serving sizes listed in the Nutrition Facts section of the labels. At first, you may want to actually measure out the amount (like 1/2 cup of ice cream or 1/4 cup of nuts) until you get used to visualizing that amount.

  We've given you examples for serving sizes on meats in the FOOD section on page 8.

- SALT—limit your intake of salt. As an alternative to regular table salt you can substitute sea salt (there's a little more nutrition in sea salt). You can spice up your food with a variety of salt-free seasonings. The longer you go without salt, the more you get used to it—it's really not such a bad deal!

15

- PLATES—try to use small plates when you eat. Your brain is easily fooled into thinking it's full when you finish the food on your small plate. If you decide you're still hungry, only take seconds on fruits and vegetables (or better yet, have another glass of water!).
- EAT—about 5 small meals a day (that means snacks are considered a meal). You need to keep your metabolism revved-up all day long—eating several small meals a day helps accomplish this.
- EXERCISE—we've touched on this before, but it's worth repeating. You don't have to join a gym (although that's not a bad idea), you don't have to buy exercise equipment—just move! Even 10 minutes a day will do wonders.

LAUGH YOUR FAT OFF

You know you're a dieter if:
- You ask how many calories are in a mint-flavored tooth pick.
- You start looking for labels on banana skins.
- You think "stow & go" means drinking lots of water.
- You accidentally park a block away from the gas station.
- Trees remind you of broccoli.
- Your favorite song is "I Like Big Butts and I Cannot Lie."
- You have your DVD set to record "Cooking with Vegetables."
- You repeatedly ask "Can I get a salad with that?"
- When someone asks "Did you get any last night?" you start counting up fruits and vegetables.
- You know that a glass of wine counts as a fruit.
- You know exactly how many calories you burn taking out the trash.
- You relieve yourself and it smells like wood chips.
- You own 2 scales, one in the bathroom and one in the kitchen.
- "Wine and Dine" becomes "Whine and Dine."

You know you're a dieter if your bumper sticker reads:
- BACK-OFF—I'M LOADED WITH FIBER!
- I've been lifting, wanna see my guns?
- I live an up-lifting life. . .at the gym.
- I brake for carrot sticks.

WORTH REPEATING

"My doctor told me to stop having intimate dinners for four. Unless there are three other people."
- Orson Welles

"There is a charm about the forbidden that makes it unspeakably desirable."
- Mark Twain

"You must begin to think of yourself as becoming the person you want to be."
- David Viscott

"Never order food in excess of your body weight."
- Erma Bombeck

"Dieting is not a piece of cake."
- Author Unknown

"You have to exercise for a week to work off the thigh fat from a single Snickers bar."
- Albert Einstein

"How long does getting thin take?"
- from Winnie the Pooh, by A.A. Milne

"I'm not overweight. I'm just nine inches too short."
- Shelley Winters

MENUS

On the next four pages you will find two week's worth of menus. These meal plans are based on 1200 calories per day. If you need to adjust these to fit your specific caloric needs (as determined by your RMR and WLCZ as computed per directions on page 12) then simply adjust the portion size for the meals or add more fruits and vegetables.

On the meal plans which follow, the items marked with an asterisk (*) have recipes provided in the Recipe section. (Sorry, we can't prepare them for you!) Additional recipes are included for your enjoyment (not to mention, variety).

You'll notice that Sunday is not included on the meal plans. It's not that we wish to eliminate the day—the reason it's not included is because you should take a day off and relax your dietary regimen for a day each week. Now, this DOESN'T mean you should eat a carton of ice cream after devouring that large pizza and anything else that fails to move out of your way! It means to relax and have fun without spending too much time fretting about what you're eating.

EAT (several small, sensible, meals a day), DRINK (lots of water) and BE HEALTHY!

	MON	TUE	WED
BREAKFAST	1 cup whole grain cereal	2 whole grain waffles	1 egg 1 slice Canadian bacon
	1 cup milk	peanut butter banana slices	1/2 whole grain English muffin
	1/2 cup fruit juice	1 cup fruit juice	
SNACK	1 medium apple 1 string cheese	1 celery stalk with 1 T. peanut butter	1 medium apple
LUNCH	*Veggie Wraps	*Twist on Tuna Salad	*Spinach Salad
			1/2 cup milk
SNACK	1 cup baby carrots	1 cup watermelon	1 cup yogurt
DINNER	*Pork Chop Skillet	*Taco Salad	*Shrimp Stir-Fry
	1 medium baked potato, 2T sour cream, 1oz cheddar cheese, 1/2 cup cooked vegetables		
	1/2 cup sugar-free pudding, 2 vanilla wafers		

THUR	FRI	SAT
*Fruit Smoothie	*Breakfast Burrito	*Veggie Omelet
1/4 cup All Bran	6 oz tomato juice	1 slice whole grain toast
protein bar	1 low-fat yogurt	8 oz protein water (i.e. K2O)
*Turkey Panini	*Fruit Plate	*Turkey Rueben
1/2 cup tomato soup		1/2 cup black beans
1/2 cup sugar-free pudding, 2 vanilla wafers	1 oz fat-free Cheddar cheese	2 cups mixed fruit
*Chicken and Rice Soup	*Chicken Enchiladas	*Quick & Thin Pizza
		*Apple Caramel Delights

	MON	TUE	WED
BREAKFAST	1 cup low-fat yogurt	1/2 cup All Bran 1/2 cup milk	*Berry Yogurt Parfait
	1 cup mixed fruit	6 oz fruit juice	
	1/4 cup granola		
SNACK	1/2 tomato 1/4 cup cottage cheese	1 banana 2 T peanut butter	6 oz tomato juice
LUNCH	*Chicken Salad on a Bed of Lettuce	Grilled Turkey Bacon Sandwich	*Barbeque Chicken Sandwich
SNACK	Small apple	baby carrots 1 T Ranch	1/2 cup pineapple
DINNER	*Lasagna	*Chicken Tacos 1/2 cup black beans	*Turkey Stroganoff 1/2 cup green beans

THUR	FRI	SAT
*Western Omelet	2 whole grain waffles	*Spinach Mushroom Enchilada
	1 T peanut butter banana slices	
celery and 2 T Low-fat cream cheese	cauliflower and 2 T ranch dressing	1/2 cup mandarin oranges
*Tuna Melt	Grilled Cheese Sandwich	Veggie Burger Baked Lays chips
	tomato soup	
1 banana 2 T peanut butter	1 kiwi	2 caramel rice cakes 1/2 cup strawberries 1/2 cup whipped topping
*Grandma's Chili	*Swedish Meatballs Over Rice	*Creole Fillets 1/2 cup rice 1/2 cup peas
1 cup frozen yogurt	1 cup mixed fruit 1/2 cup whipped topping	

Recipes:
Breakfast:
- Fruit Smoothie
- Breakfast Burrito
- Veggie Omelet
- Berry Yogurt Parfait
- Western Omelet
- Spinach Mushroom Enchilada

Lunch:
- Veggie Wraps
- A Twist on Tuna
- Spinach Salad
- Turkey Panini
- Fruit Plate
- Turkey Reuben
- Chicken Salad on a Bed of Lettuce
- Barbeque Chicken Sandwich
- Tuna Melt

Dinner:
- Pork Chop Skillet
- Taco Salad
- Shrimp Stir-Fry
- Chicken and Rice Soup
- Chicken Enchiladas
- Quick & Thin Pizza
- Lasagna
- Chicken Tacos
- Turkey Stroganoff
- Grandma's Chili
- Swedish Meatballs over Rice
- Creole Fillets

Desserts:
- Apple Caramel Delights
- Chocolate Cake Brownies
- Berry Trifle
- Strawberry Pie
- Carrot Cake Bars

Lunch Options:
400 calories each
- Half Turkey Sandwich and Soup
- Half Chicken Sandwich with Baked Potato
- Tuna on Crackers with Sweet Potato
- Peanut Butter and Jelly Sandwich
- Half Grilled Cheese Sandwich and Soup
- Turkey Breast Sandwich with Orange

Extras:
- No Time for Breakfast
- Fake Fried Chicken
- Walleye Fish Cakes
- Broccoli Cheese Soup
- Turkey Burrito Roll Up
- Light & Crispy Pizza

100 Calorie Snack Ideas

Abbreviations:
tsp = teaspoon
Tbls = tablespoon
pkg = package

Fruit Smoothie:
Serves: 2
150 cal

1 banana
1 cup pineapple
1/2 cup raspberries
1 cup Orange Juice
1 ½ cups crushed ice

1. Add fruit to blender and mix on light for one minute.
2. Add juice and ice.
3. Mix on light for one minute.
4. Serve.

Breakfast Burrito
Serves: 4
370 calories

1 cup frozen hashbrowns
1/4 cup chopped onion
1 tsp olive oil
1 cup Egg Beaters or 2 whole eggs plus 2 egg whites
1/8 tsp black pepper
4 whole wheat tortillas warmed
1/3 cup shredded low fat cheddar cheese
1/2 cup salsa

1. In large nonstick skillet, sauté, over medium heat, potatoes and onion in 1 tsp olive oil until tender.
2. Add egg and sprinkle with pepper.
3. Cook, stirring occasionally, until eggs are set.
4. Divide mixture evenly between tortillas.
5. Top with cheese and salsa.
6. Serve.

Veggie Omelet

Serves: 3
250 calories

1/4 cup sliced portabella mushrooms
1 cup chopped broccoli
1/3 cup chopped onion
1/4 cup red pepper
1 tsp minced garlic
5 tsp extra virgin olive oil
3/4 cup low-fat cottage cheese
1/4 cup low-fat shredded mozzarella
3 egg beaters
1/3 cup chopped tomato

1. In non-stick skillet heat 2 tsp olive oil over medium heat.
2. Sauté broccoli, mushrooms, onion, red pepper and garlic until tender.
3. Remove from heat.
4. Pour veggie combo into mixing bowl and add cottage cheese.
5. In the same skillet, heat 1 tsp olive oil over medium heat.
6. Pour in 1 of the egg beaters.
7. Cook until eggs are set.
8. Add 1/3 cup veggies mix to 1/2 side of omelet and fold uncovered side over veggies.
9. Top with mozzarella cheese and 1 Tbsp tomatoes.
10. Repeat recipe to complete all three omelets.

Berry Yogurt Parfait

200 calories
Serves: 4

2 cups low-fat vanilla yogurt
1 cup strawberries
1/2 cup blueberries
1 cup low-fat granola

1. Combine yogurt and fruit in mixing bowl.
2. Top with granola and serve.

Western Omelet
Serves: 1
219 calories

1/2 cup diced potatoes
2 slices turkey bacon, chopped
1/2 cup chopped red and green bell peppers
2 tsp extra-virgin olive oil
1 cup Egg Beaters
1/4 cup chopped green onions

1. In 8 inch skillet over medium heat, sauté potatoes, bell pepper, turkey bacon and onion in 1 tsp olive oil until tender.
2. Remove from skillet.
3. In same skillet, add 1 tsp olive oil.
4. Pour Egg Beaters into skillet.
5. Cook until egg is almost set.
6. Add veggie mixture over half of omelet.
7. Fold uncovered half over mixture and serve.

Spinach Mushroom Enchilada
180 Calories
Serves: 8

1/2 cup sliced mushrooms
2 pkg (10 OZ EACH) frozen chopped spinach
2 cup ricotta cheese
1 tsp salt
1/4 tsp pepper
8-8 inch whole wheat tortillas
1 cup shredded lettuce
1 cup dice tomatoes

1. Combine mushrooms and spinach.
2. Sauté over medium heat until heated thoroughly.
3. Divide spinach filling into 8 portions.
4. Spoon onto center of tortillas.
5. Roll tortillas and place in 12x8 microwavable dish.
6. Microwave tortillas at medium heat for 10 minutes.
7. Sprinkle with cheese. Reheat tortillas until cheese is melted.
8. Sprinkle enchilada with lettuce and tomatoes and serve.

Veggie Wraps:
Serves 4
293 calories

4 whole wheat tortillas (8-inch)
1 cup fat-free cottage cheese
1/4 cup tomatoes, diced
1/4 cup yellow bell peppers, diced
1/8 cup green onions, diced
1/4 tsp lemon juice
1/8 tsp garlic salt
Black pepper to taste
4 leaves lettuce

1. Combine cottage cheese, tomato, yellow pepper and green onion together.
2. Add lemon juice and seasoning. Blend.
3. Place leaf lettuce on tortilla and top with 1/3 cup cottage cheese and veggies.
4. Roll and serve.

A Twist on Tuna
Serves: 4
Calories: 258

1 can or pkg water-packed Tuna
2 Tbls light mayo
1/2 medium apple, chopped
1/2 stalk celery, chopped
1/4 cup walnuts, chopped
4 lettuce leaf
2 whole grain bagels

1. In mixing bowl combine tuna, mayo, apple, celery and walnuts.
2. Place one leaf lettuce on each one-half of bagel.
3. Divide tuna mixture evenly between bagel halves.
4. Serve.

Spinach Salad
Serves 1
300 calories

2 cups spinach
1 Tbls low-fat ranch dressing
1 ounce chicken breast sliced
2 Tbls sliced almonds
1/4 cup mandarin oranges

1. Place spinach in a serving bowl.
2. Top with sliced chicken.
3. Top with mandarin oranges.
4. Top with sliced almonds.
5. Mix in ranch dressing.
6. Serve.

Turkey Panini
Serves: 1
275 calories

2 slices Panini bread
1 ounce sliced turkey
1 Tbls light mayo
1 Tbls barbeque sauce
3/4 ounce cheddar cheese
1 tsp butter

1. Butter one side of both pieces of bread.
2. Place one piece of bread on flat pan sprayed with olive oil cooking spray.
3. Top with turkey and cheese.
4. Combine light mayo and barbeque sauce in small mixing dish.
5. Spread mixture on opposite side of buttered bread.
6. Place bread on top of turkey and cheese.
7. Brown both sides of sandwich until golden.
8. Serve.

Fruit Plate
Serves: 1
300 calories

1 cup low-fat cottage cheese
1/4 cup pineapple
1/4 cup cantaloupe
2 stems grapes, stems removed

1. Place 1 cup of cottage cheese on small serving plate.
2. Top with fruit.
3. Serve chilled.

Turkey Rueben
Serves: 4
400 calories

3 Tbls butter
8 slices rye bread
3 Tbls low-fat Thousand Island dressing
6 oz thinly sliced turkey
4 slices low-fat Swiss cheese
1 cup low-sodium sauerkraut

1. Spread butter on one side of each bread slice and salad dressing on the other with the butter side down.
2. Top four slices of bread with meat, cheese and sauerkraut.
3. Top with remaining bread slices, dressing side down.
4. Preheat large skillet over medium heat.
5. Reduce heat to medium-low.
6. Cook for 4 to 6 minutes or until bread is toasted and cheese is melted. Turn once.
7. Serve.

Chicken Salad on a Bed of Lettuce
Serves 4
266 calories

3 boneless skinless chicken breasts
6 green onions
4 shredded carrots
1/4 cup shredded low-fat cheddar cheese
1/4 cup light mayo

1. Cook chicken according to package directions.
2. In a separate bowl mix together onions, carrots, cheese and mayo.
3. Once chicken is thoroughly cooked, shred chicken and add to mayo mixture.
4. Serve on a bed of lettuce or bread of choice (calories listed are for salad mixtures and do not include bread).

Barbeque Chicken Sandwich
Serves 4
450 calories

1 Tbls paprika
1 tsp onion powder
1 tsp cayenne pepper
1 tsp black pepper
4 skinless chicken breast halves
4 slices low-fat mozzarella cheese
1/4 cup low-fat mayo
8 slices whole wheat bread

1. Mix together paprika, onion powder, cayenne pepper and black pepper.
2. Rub chicken breasts with seasoning mixture until breast is fully coated.
3. Preheat flat pan on medium-high heat.
4. Lightly spray pan with olive oil cooking spray.
5. Place chicken on pan and cook for 6 to 8 minutes on each side until chicken is fully cooked (can be done on grill also).
6. Place cheese slice on top of each breast.
7. Cook until cheese is melted.
8. Place a chicken breast on a slice of bread. Repeat for each chicken breast.
9. Spread 1 Tbls of low-fat mayo onto remaining slices of bread and place mayo-side down on top of sandwiches.

Tuna Melt
Serves 4
239 calories

1 pkg tuna packed in water
2 Tbls chopped onion
2 Tbls pickled relish
1/4 cup light mayo
4 slices Swiss cheese
4 slices whole grain bread

1. Toast bread slices.
2. Mix together tuna, onion, relish and mayo.
3. Spread tuna mixture on toasted bread slices.
4. Top with cheese.
5. Broil 4 to 5 minutes or until cheese is fully melted and serve.

Pork Chop Skillet
Serves: 4
235 calories

4 (6 oz) pork chops
1 tsp olive oil
1/4 cup balsamic vinaigrette dressing
1 small onion, sliced
1 tsp garlic minced

1. Brown chops in olive oil in nonstick skillet over medium to high heat. Remove chops from skillet and set aside.
2. Add 2 Tbls of vinaigrette dressing, onion and garlic. Cook for 4 minutes.
3. Add chops to skillet and remaining 2 Tbls of dressing.
4. Simmer on medium to low heat for 10 minutes or until pork chops are thoroughly cooked.
5. Serve.

Taco Salad

Serves 4
367 calories

1 lb ground turkey
1 package taco seasoning mix
1/3 can black beans, drained
1/3 cup low-fat ranch salad dressing
1 cup chopped lettuce
1 medium chopped tomato
1 small chopped onion
1 small can sliced black olives
1/2 cup salsa
1-1/3 cup shredded low-fat cheddar cheese

1. Brown ground turkey in large skillet. Cook over medium heat until meat is fully cooked.
2. Drain excess fat.
3. Stir in taco seasoning mix and black beans.
4. Simmer for 5 minutes.
5. Remove from heat and set aside.
6. Place lettuce in serving dish, top with meat mixture.
7. Top with chopped tomato, onion and black olives.
8. In a mixing bowl combine salsa and ranch dressing.
9. Top salad with salsa mixture and cheese.
10. Serve.

Shrimp Stir-Fry

Serves: 4

395 calories

3 cups whole grain rice
3/4 cup reduced sodium chicken broth
1 Tbls cornstarch
1 Tbsp Tamari—low-sodium
1 tsp red wine vinegar
1 tsp sugar
2 tsp olive oil
1 small onion, wedged
1 tsp garlic, minced
1/2 lb medium shrimp, peeled and deveined
2 cups green peas

1. Cook rice as directed and set aside.
2. Blend broth, cornstarch, tamari, red wine vinegar and sugar in small mixing bowl until smooth.
3. Heat oil in large nonstick skillet over medium heat until hot.
4. Add onion and garlic.
5. Stir fry 2 to 3 minutes.
6. Add shrimp and green peas.
7. Stir chicken broth mixture and add to skillet.
8. Cook 1 minute or until boiling.
9. Serve over rice.

Chicken and Rice Soup

Serves: 3
153 calories

1 cup uncooked brown rice
3—10 ¾ oz cans reduced sodium chicken broth
1 skinless, diced chicken breast
1 stalk celery, chopped
1 carrot, sliced
1/4 cup onion, chopped
2 tsp ground parsley
1/4 tsp thyme
1/8 tsp pepper

1. Cook rice as directed on package and set aside.
2. Combine in a separate saucepan broth and chicken.
3. Bring to a boil.
4. Reduce heat and simmer 10 minutes.
5. Add celery, carrot, onion and parsley.
6. Simmer 10 minutes or until chicken is thoroughly cooked and vegetables are tender.
7. Add rice, thyme and pepper to saucepan.
8. Cook over medium heat 8 minutes.
9. Serve.

Chicken Enchiladas
Serves: 4
545 calories

3 chicken breasts
1 cup low-fat cheddar cheese
1 cup low-fat sour cream
1 can black beans
2 cans chopped tomatoes with green chilies
10 wheat tortillas
2 Tbls low-fat mozzarella cheese

1. Grill chicken until thoroughly cooked. Dice.
2. Blend chicken, 1/2 cup cheddar cheese, sour cream, beans and tomatoes in a mixing bowl.
3. Cut tortillas into strips.
4. Line baking dish with strips.
5. Spoon in ½ of the chicken mixture on top of tortilla strips.
6. Layer strips again.
7. Top with remaining chicken mixture.
8. Top with ½ cup of cheese.
9. Bake at 350 for 1 hr.
10. Sprinkle with mozzarella cheese.
11. Cover and bake for 30 minutes.

Quick and Thin Pizza
Serves 1
Cal 250

1 8 inch flour tortilla
1/4 cup Light Ragu tomato basil spaghetti sauce
1/4 cup Sliced mushrooms
1 slice Swiss cheese

1. Heat broiler to 500 degrees.
2. Spread Ragu on tortilla.
3. Top with mushrooms.
4. Broil 2 to 3 minutes until bubbly.
5. Top with cheese and broil until cheese is melted.

Lasagna
676 calories
Serves: 3

1 lb ground turkey
2 cups low-sodium spaghetti sauce
1 can sliced mushrooms (drained)
1 Tbls garlic powder
1 ½ tsp oregano
6 cooked lasagna noodles (according to pkg. directions)
1/2 cup low-fat Ricotta Cheese
6 Tbls low-fat Parmesan Cheese
3/4 cup low-fat Mozzarella Cheese

1. Preheat oven to 350 degrees.
2. Brown ground turkey in large nonstick skillet.
3. Drain any excess fat.
4. Add spaghetti sauce, mushrooms, garlic and oregano.
5. Bring to boil.
6. Reduce heat.
7. Simmer uncovered for 8 minutes.
8. Spray 8 inch square baking dish with vegetable oil.
9. Place 2 noodles on bottom of pan. Cover with 1/3 of the turkey/sauce mix, then 1/3 of the various cheeses.
10. Layer remaining noodles and sauce, topping each layer with the various cheeses.
11. Bake for 45 minutes or until cheese is lightly browned.

Chicken Tacos
Serves 4
292 calories

4 chicken breasts
1/2 jar salsa
1/2 pkg taco seasoning
4 taco shells

1. Place chicken breasts in bottom of crock pot.
2. Top with salsa and seasoning mix.
3. Cook on low for 8 hours.
4. Shred and serve in taco shells.

Turkey Stroganoff

Serves 4

470 Calories

1 lb ground turkey
1 can low-sodium beef broth
1 cup water
1/2 package wide egg noodles
1 can sliced mushrooms
1 can low-fat cream of mushroom soup
1 cup low-fat sour cream

1. Brown turkey and drain.
2. Add beef broth, water, noodles and mushrooms to skillet.
3. Bring to boil and continue to boil until noodles are tender and liquid is almost gone.
4. Add cream of mushroom soup and sour cream.
5. Simmer for 5 minutes.
6. Remove from heat and serve.

Grandma's Chili

Serves: 4

313 calories

1 lb ground turkey
2 (12 ounce) cans tomato juice
1 med onion, chopped
1 packet taco seasoning mix
2 (15 ounce) cans regular chili beans

1. In large nonstick skillet brown turkey until thoroughly cooked.
2. Lower heat and drain any excess fat.
3. Add tomato juice, onion, and taco seasoning.
4. Stir. Add chili beans, stirring frequently.
5. Let simmer 10 minutes.
6. If desired, top with diced tomatoes, shredded lettuce, sliced black olives, and low-fat cheese. (Add 30 calories for each 1/4 cup cheese.)

Swedish Meatballs over Rice

Serves: 4

370 Calories

2 ½ cups whole grain rice
1 lb lean ground beef
1/8 tsp seasoning salt
1/8 tsp garlic salt
1/8 tsp black pepper
1/4 cup finely chopped onion
2 tsp olive oil
1/2 cup flour
1 can low-fat cream of mushroom soup
3/4 cup low-fat sour cream
1 Tbls Worcestershire Sauce

1. Cook rice according to package directions, set aside.
2. In a mixing bowl combine beef, ½ cup rice, seasoning salt, garlic salt, pepper and onion together.
3. In nonstick skillet heat oil on medium heat.
4. Roll beef mixture into medium size balls (should make about 20 meatballs).
5. Roll balls in flour and place in skillet.
6. Cook beef balls until browned.
7. In separate bowl mix soup, sour cream and Worcestershire sauce.
8. Pour soup mixture over meatballs and simmer 30 minutes.
9. Serve over remaining rice.

Creole Fillets
Serves: 6
293 Calories

1 c chopped onion
1 c chopped green pepper
1 clove garlic, minced
3 T olive oil
2-1 lb cans tomatoes
1 or 2 bay leaves
1 ½ t. salt
Cayenne pepper to taste
2 lbs frozen halibut

1. Cook onion, pepper, and garlic in 3 T olive oil until tender.
2. Add tomatoes, bay leaf, salt and dash of cayenne.
3. Simmer 30 minutes.
4. Place frozen fish in 11 x 7 baking dish, sprinkle with salt and pepper.
5. Pour tomato mixture over fish.
6. Bake at 350 degrees for 45 minutes.

Apple Caramel Delights
Serves: 1
106 calories

2 Quaker caramel corn rice cakes
1 tsp caramel syrup
1 cup fat-free whipped topping
1 apple thinly sliced

1. Spread whipped topping onto rice cakes.
2. Top with apples.
3. Drizzle caramel syrup.
4. Serve.

Chocolate Cake Brownies

Serves: 9
Calories: 215

2 oz. unsweetened chocolate, chopped
2 Tbls vegetable oil (sunflower or safflower)
3/4 cup All Bran cereal
1/2 cup low-fat buttermilk
2 large eggs, plus 2 egg whites
2 tsp vanilla
1 cup grated zucchini
1/2 cup unsweetened cocoa powder
3/4 cup sugar
1/4 cup unbleached flour
1/2 tsp baking soda
1/4 tsp salt
2 Tbls powdered sugar (if desired)

1. Preheat oven to 350 degrees.
2. Combine chocolate and vegetable oil in microwaveable bowl.
3. Microwave on high 1 1/2 to 2 minutes.
4. Stir until smooth. Let cool.
5. Pour cereal into a food processor, add buttermilk, and pulse until cereal is finely ground.
6. Scrape down side of food processor and let mixture stand for 15 minutes.
7. Add eggs, vanilla, zucchini, and melted chocolate—pulse until blended.
8. Sift cocoa over a large bowl, to remove any lumps, add sugar, flour, baking soda, and salt. Stir with a wire whisk.
9. Stir in cereal mixture.
10. Pour into 9-inch square baking pan sprayed with vegetable oil.
11. Bake 30 to 33 minutes, until toothpick inserted in center comes out with a few moist crumbs attached.
12. Cool completely.
13. Sift powdered sugar over to serve, if desired.

Berry Trifle
Serves: 15
Calories: 210

1 15 oz. carton low-fat ricotta cheese
1 8 oz. low-fat lemon or vanilla yogurt
7 Tbls powdered sugar
2 tsp vanilla
1 10-inch commercial angle food cake, cut into 1 in. cubes
1 medium banana
2 tsp lemon juice
2 cup frozen, thawed raspberries
2 cup fresh or frozen thawed blueberries
2 cup sliced fresh strawberries
1 ½ cup light whipped topping, thawed

1. In a blender, combine ricotta, yogurt, powdered sugar and vanilla. Process until smooth.
2. Layer 1/3 of the cake cubes in bottom of deep serving bowl.
3. Spoon 1/3 of ricotta mixture over cake.
4. Slice banana and toss in lemon juice.
5. Layer 1/3 each of banana, raspberries and blueberries over ricotta.
6. Repeat 2 more times.
7. Spread with whipped topping and chill about 2 hours before serving.

Strawberry Pie
Serves: 8
Calories: 160

4 oz strawberry gelatin
2/3 cup boiling water
1/2 cup cold water
Ice cubes
8 oz. Light whipped topping
3/4 cup sliced strawberries
1/4 cup pineapple tidbits in juice, drained and dried
 1 graham cracker pie crust

1. Pour gelatin into large bowl.
2. Pour boiling water over gelatin and stir until dissolved.
3. Pour 1/2 cup cold water into 4 cup measuring cup, add ice cubes to make 1 1/4 cup.
4. Pour gelatin into cold water and mix until it thickens.
5. Stir in 3 1/2 cup whipped topping, mix until smooth.
6. Fold in fruit and mix lightly.
7. Refrigerate mixture 3 to 4 hours until thickened.
8. Pour into pie shell and top with additional topping, if desired.

Carrot Cake Bars

Serves: 20
Calories: 120

3/4 cup unbleached flour
1/4 cup honey
1/4 cup whole wheat flour
1 1/2 tsp pumpkin pie spice
1 tsp baking powder
1/8 tsp salt
1 cup finely shredded carrots
3/4 cup chopped walnuts or pecans
3 egg whites, lightly beaten
1/4 cup cooking oil (sunflower or safflower)
1/4 cup low-fat milk

1. Preheat oven to 350 degrees.
2. Line 9x9x2 inch baking pan with foil, lightly coat with cooking spray
3. In medium bowl, combine both flours, pumpkin pie spice, baking powder, and salt.
4. Add carrots, honey, eggs, oil and milk and 1/2 of nuts.
5. Stir until combined.
6. Spread evenly in foil-lined pan.
7. Bake 15 to 18 minutes, or until toothpick inserted in middle comes out clean.
8. Cool on wire rack.
9. Holding onto foil, lift uncut bars from pan.
10. Turn upside down onto serving plate.
11. Spread frosting evenly.
12. Sprinkle with remaining nuts.
13. Cut into 20 bars.

FROSTING:
1/2 cup light whipped topping, thawed
4 oz. reduced-fat cream cheese
1/4 cup low-fat vanilla yogurt

1. In medium bowl, beat cream cheese until smooth.
2. Add yogurt, beat until smooth.
3. Fold in thawed whipped topping.

Half Turkey Sandwich with Soup
Serves: 1
400 calories

1 slice whole wheat bread
1 oz turkey lunch meat
3/4 oz cheddar cheese
1 Tbls light mayo
1/2 cup corn
1 tsp butter
1/2 cup tomato soup

Half Chicken Sandwich with Baked Potato
Serves: 1
400 calories

1 slice whole wheat bread
1 oz baked skinless chicken breast
3/4 oz cheddar cheese
1 Tbls light mayo
1/2 cup baked potato
2 tsp butter
3 tsp sour cream

Tuna Salad on Crackers with Sweet Potato
Serves: 1
400 calories

5 whole wheat crackers
1 oz light tuna canned in water
1 Tbls light mayo
1/2 cup sweet potato
2 tsp butter
1/2 cup chocolate 1% fat milk

Peanut Butter and Jelly Sandwich
Serves: 1
400 calories

2 slices whole wheat bread
1 Tbls Peanut Butter
2 Tbls Jelly
1/2 cup skim milk

Half Grilled Cheese Sandwich and Soup
Serves 1
400 calories

1 slice whole wheat bread
3/4 oz cheddar cheese
2 tsp margarine
1/2 cup low-sodium chicken noodle soup

Turkey Breast Sandwich with Orange
Serves: 1
400 calories

2 slices whole wheat bread
2 oz low-sodium turkey breast
1 oz cheese
1 Tbls mustard
lettuce
tomato
1 orange

No Time for Breakfast
Serves: 2
200 Calories

2 low-fat, whole grain waffles
2/3 cup sugar-free cherry pie filling
    or sugar-free apple pie filling, divided
2 Tbls low-fat yogurt

1. Toast the waffles in toaster.
2. Top with 1/3 cup pie filling and 1 Tbls yogurt.

Fake Fried Chicken
Serves: 6
185 Calories

olive oil cooking spray
6 whole boneless, skinless chicken breast halves
1 ¾ cup cold water
1/2 cup plain non-fat yogurt

Breading Mix:
1/2 cup flour
1/2 Tbls Herb and Garlic Old Bay Seasoning
1/8 tsp black pepper
1/4 tsp Cajun seasoning
1/4 tsp thyme
1/4 tsp oregano
1/2 cup Italian-seasoned bread crumbs

1. Preheat oven to 400 degrees.
2. Coat a baking sheet with olive oil cooking spray.
3. Place chicken in large bowl of very cold water.
4. Dump yogurt into a medium mixing bowl and set aside.
5. Place breading ingredients into a sealed mixing bag and shake well to mix.
6. Remove 1 piece of chicken from bowl and roll in yogurt.
7. Place chicken breast in bag and shake to coat.
8. Place coated chicken onto baking sheet.
9. Repeat steps for all 6 chicken breasts.
10. Bake 1 hour, turning breasts every 20 minutes to allow for thorough cooking.
11. Serve.

Walleye Fish Cakes
Serves: 4
65 calories

1 celery stalk
1 yellow squash
2 medium onions
18 oz walleye
6 Tbls Italian-seasoned bread crumbs
2 large eggs
1/4 tsp black pepper
1 tsp garlic salt

1. Wash, peel, and chop all vegetables and dump into large mixing bowl.
2. Cut walleye in small pieces and add to bowl.
3. In separate bowl, mix together bread crumbs, eggs, pepper, and garlic salt.
4. Dump egg mixture into bowl with fish and stir.
5. With a large mixing spoon create small cakes and place them in nonstick skillet.
6. Cover and cook on medium heat for 5-7 minutes, then turn over to brown on both sides.
7. Serve.

Broccoli & Cheese Soup
Serves: 12
150 calories

4 Tbls butter
3/4 cup chopped onion
1/2 cup flour
4 cups low-sodium chicken broth
4 cups 1% milk
16 oz frozen chopped broccoli
2 cups raw diced potatoes
1 Tbls Worcestershire
1/2 tsp pepper
1 ½ cups low-fat cheddar cheese

1. Melt butter in saucepan over medium heat.
2. Add onion and cook until tender.
3. Add flour stirring continuously.
4. Stir in broth slowly.
5. Add milk, broccoli and potatoes. Cook 15 minutes over low heat until vegetables are tender.
6. Stir in Worcestershire, pepper and cheese.
7. Cook until cheese is melted.

Turkey Burrito Roll Up

Serves: 4
500 calories

1/2 lb. ground turkey
2 tsp chili powder
1 can (15 oz.) black beans, drained, rinsed
1/2 cup chunky salsa
3/4 cup shredded reduced-fat sharp cheddar cheese
4 flour tortillas (10 inch)
1/4 cup reduced-fat or light sour cream
1 tomato, chopped
1 cup shredded romaine lettuce

1. Cook turkey and chili powder in large skillet on medium heat until meat is thoroughly cooked.
2. Add beans and salsa. Cook 5 minutes or until heated through, stirring occasionally.
3. Remove from heat. Stir in cheese.
4. Spread meat mixture down centers of tortillas. Top with sour cream, tomatoes and lettuce.
5. Roll up burrito-style.

Light and Crispy Pizza

Serves: 1

250 Calories

1 low-fat whole wheat tortilla
1/2 Tbls ranch dressing
1/8 tsp garlic powder
1/4 cup diced red, yellow, and green peppers
5 black olives, sliced
2-3 sliced mushrooms
1/4 cup low-fat shredded mozzarella cheese

1. Preheat oven to 425°F.
2. Place wheat tortilla on a baking sheet and place in preheated oven for 3 minutes, then flip tortilla and toast for another 2-3 minutes until tortilla is browned on both sides.
3. Remove from oven and immediately top with Ranch Dressing and garlic powder.
4. Add the peppers, olives and mushrooms and top with mozzarella cheese.
5. Bake for about 5 minutes or until cheese is melted.
6. Serve.

100 Calorie or Less Snack Ideas:

1 large stalk celery with 1 Tbls peanut butter or 1 Tbls cream cheese

1 large dill pickle wrapped in 1 slice ham and 1 slice Swiss cheese

1/2 cup Frosted Mini Wheat cereal

1 medium banana

1/2 cup applesauce

1 cup grapes

2 cups watermelon

2 slices bacon

2 Tbls sunflower seeds

1/3 cup sherbet

1/2 cup frozen yogurt

8 m&m's

1 oz jelly beans